CHILDREN

COLDS:

40 NATURAL REMEDIES

Practical Guide

J. R. R. Perkins

Table of Content

Chapter 1: What is a cold?

A cold is a viral infection that affects the upper respiratory tract (nose, throat, and sinuses), being more common during the autumn and winter months or when significant changes in temperature unfold. Colds can last between three and eleven days and they are the most common illness among children and adults of all ages, being the main reason to consult with a pediatric.

Healthy children (except babies) can suffer around eight colds during the fall and winter months, as they are in contact with other children and their bodies are still developing their defenses. With the pass of the years, children develop a repertoire of anti-virus that proportionate immunity against colds and help their bodies to confront infections.

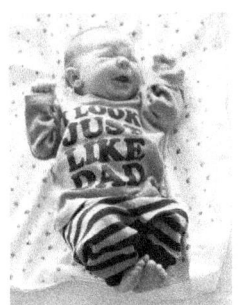

4

There are more than 200 different viruses that could be involved in a cold but the most common one is the rhinovirus.

As colds are viral infections, antibiotics will not improve the symptoms. All the opposite, antibiotics will only weaken the body, making it more vulnerable to the attack of another virus.

During the early stages of a cold, your child may complain of headaches and congestion. As the cold progresses, the mucus secretions from the sinuses may turn darker and thicker and mild cough could be developed.

Sometimes side effects associated with a cold, like stress or fatigue, can cause bacterial infections that will require the attention of a qualified doctor.

Typical cold symptoms include:

- Runny or stuffed-up nose that lasts up to 10 days;
- Cough;
- Headache;
- Mild sore throat (2 or 3 weeks);

- Loss of appetite;

- Fatigue;

- Ear pain;

- Inflammation of the ganglions (on the neck);

- Crying eyes;

- Diarrhea and vomiting (on occasions);

- Mild fever (on occasion- 2 or 3 days)

Chapter 2: How do colds spread?

Children can catch colds from members of the family, pets, teachers, babysitters, other children, and even objects.

The contagion could be direct (kissing, touching or holding hands with an infected person), indirect (by touching a toy, a tissue, etc. that has been touched by an infected person) or through air pollution (most germs spread when a person coughs or sneezes).

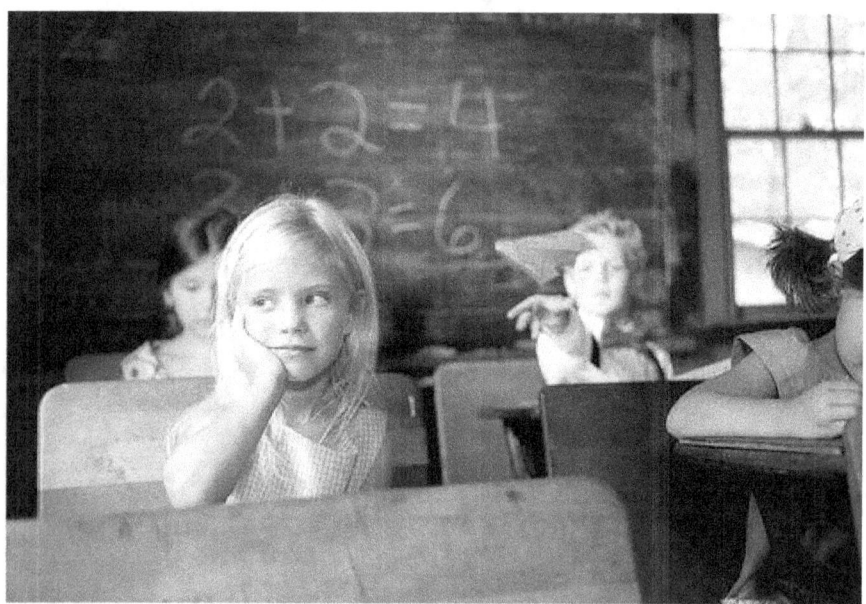

Different statistics confirm that a young child can get as many as 10 colds before he reaches the age of 2. In fact, statistics show that preschool-aged children have around 9 colds per year, kindergartners can have 12 colds per year and teenagers and adults have around 7 colds on an annual basis.

Chapter 3: What to do when your child gets a cold?

There is no cure for the common cold and it usually goes away on its own. However, they are a number of tips that will help your child go through the process:

- Keep your child as comfortable as possible.

- Make him drink a lot of caffeine-free fluids to keep the body hydrated, which will help the organism to confront the effects of a cold. Children between the ages of 3 months and 1 year should take between one and three teaspoons of warm liquids like water, apple juice, etc. four times a day. If your child is younger than 3 months, medical attention is required.

- Feed your child with small and nutritious meals.

- Keep the temperature of the child's room between 18 and 22° C and check your child's temperature constantly.

- Do not give acetylsalicylic acid (Aspirin) to children with colds because it can derive in cases of brain and liver damage (Reye syndrome- a rare disorder that occurs in children under 15) and whatever you do never medicate your child with over-the-counter cold medicines, especially when you child is younger than 6 years old. Instead, consult your pharmacist or even better, your doctor.

- Although a humidifier in your child's bedroom at night will help him breathe, its use should be limited, as cool mist humidifiers can present a risk of contamination from bacteria and mold while hot water vaporizers are not recommended because of the risk of burns.

- Children can continue their normal activities and daily lives if they feel well enough to do so.

Call your doctor to make an appointment or take your child to an emergency department if you notice your child:

- Is breathing rapidly or seems to be working hard to breathe, sleep or eat;

- Breathes more than 60 breathes per minute in babies and more than 40 in children over two years old;

- Has blue lips;

- Looks too weak or it is very difficult to wake him;

- Presents signs of dehydration or has diarrhea and vomits;

- Has a fever for more than 3 days or over 38° C;

- Has a fever and he is younger than 3 months old;

- Is coughing so bad that he is choking or vomiting;

- Wakes in the morning with one or both eyes stuck shut with dried yellow pus;

- Is much more sleepy than usual and does not want to play or eat and cannot be comforted;

- Presents signs of ear infection;

- Has yellow or green discharge through the eyes;

- Has a cough for more than 3 weeks or sore throat for more than 24 hours;

- Has thick or colored (yellow, green) discharge from the nose for more than 10 to 14 days;

- o Symptoms have not improved in a week;

- o Fever returns in the middle of the cold or increases suddenly;

- o The child shows signs of pain or pulls his ears

Do not ignore the symptoms, as some respiratory viruses can derive in serious illnesses like bronchitis or pneumonia.

Chapter 4: How to prevent colds?

It is basically impossible to avoid colds when there is a child at home and it is very possible that the entire family and pets end up suffering the effects of the cold.

The common cold virus can spread quickly through the air and it can stay for hours on hand-touched objects such as stair railings, books, door handles, computers, toys, etc.

There are a series of useful tips that can drastically reduce the chances of getting contagious:

- Teach your child to wash his hands after every bathroom trip; before every meal; after being in contact with someone who shows cold symptoms; after coughing, sneezing or wiping his nose and after playing at school or at home. Children should wash their hands with warm soapy water.

- Keep your child at home to avoid passing the cold to other children at school.

- Teach your child to cover his mouth when sneezing or coughing and to use a tissue for nose blowing.

- Wash your own hands and your child's hands after wiping your child's nose.

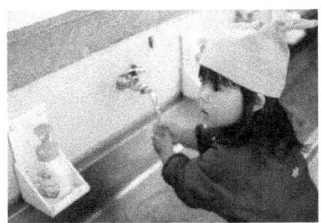

- Keep babies under 3 months old away from people with colds, if possible.

- Teach your child to not share toys that young children place in their mouths until they have been cleaned.

- Teach your child to avoid sharing cups, utensils, pacifiers or towels with others.

- Teach your child to avoid kissing people with cold symptoms.

- Refresh the child's room frequently.

- Feed your child with food rich in vitamin C like citric, tomatoes, and fresh vegetables.

- Avoid close contact with smokers, as the smoke could worsen breathing problems.

- Prevent colds by offering your child supplements like Zinc or multivitamins.

Chapter 5: What is the difference between cold and influenza?

Influenza (or "flu") is a respiratory infection caused by influenza virus. Like a cold, the months of autumn and winter are the ones linked to major influenza offspring.

Differently from the cold, the virus of influenza becomes stronger and immune, and this means that from time to time, there is a major mutation in the influenza virus and no one is immune.

Influenza viruses affect the respiratory system and it can be passed from one person to another through the air, through hand-caught objects, and through direct contact with affected people.

The flu strikes quicker than a cold and its typical symptoms include:

- Sudden fever, even over 39° C;
- Stomach pain;

- Vomiting and/or diarrhea;

- Chills and shakes;

- Headaches;

- Muscle aches and inflammation (occasionally, 2-4 days);

- Extreme fatigue (up to 2 weeks);

- Back pain;

- Dry cough;

- Sore throat;

- Ear pain;

- Red eyes;

- Loss of appetite

Chapter 6: What to do against influenza?

- Keep your child as comfortable as possible.

- Try to make sure your kid ingests plenty of fluids.

- Feed your child small and nutritious meals.

- In case of fever, dress the child with lightweight clothing (preferably just underwear) and keep the room temperature around 20°C.

- Gargling with warm water will ease a sore throat. For children 3 years or older who can safely suck on hard candy without choking, you can offer them sugarless hard candies or lozenges containing honey, herbs or pectin.

- Check your child's temperature. To ease pain, aches or a fever use Ibuprofen when the child is over 6 months old, after checking with your doctor.

- Unless your doctor says otherwise, give the dose recommended on the package every 4 hours until the child's temperature comes down.

- Do not give acetylsalicylic acid (Aspirin) to children with colds because it can derive in cases of brain and liver damage (Reye syndrome- a rare disorder that occurs in children under 15) and whatever you do never medicate your child with over-the-counter cold medicines, especially when you child is younger than 6 years old. The *American Academy of Pediatrics* warns that over-the-counter medications are not safe for children under 2 and may not work or could seriously harm children under 6. Instead, consult your pharmacist or even better, your doctor.

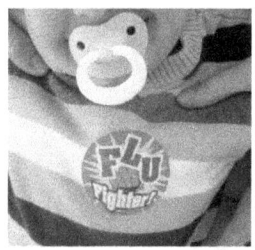

19

Influenza can lead to bacterial infections of the ear (otitis), lung (pneumonia), sinuses (sinusitis), and even serious conditions like pneumonia or bronchitis.

In rare cases, influenza can affect the brain, heart or weaken the immune system. Call your doctor or take your child to an emergency department if he:

- Has problems breathing (rapidly or hard breathe);
- Is not eating and/or drinking or is vomiting for more than 4 hours or has diarrhea;
- Has a fever over 38°C or higher;
- Has chest pain or severe cough;
- Coughing so bad that he is choking or vomiting;
- Has not urinated at least every 6 hours when awake;
- Feels more sleepy than usual or is unable to move;
- Refuses to play and eat and cannot be comforted;
- Is not feeling better after 5 days or was feeling better and suddenly is sick again;
- Has blue lips;

- Shows febrile convulsions or seems confused;

- Has a stiff neck

- Shows signs of the flu and has a serious chronic illness;

- Has been coughing for more than a week.

Chapter 7: How to prevent influenza?

- Children over 6 months old should get vaccinated against flu every year, especially children who are at high risk of complications from influenza. Therefore, you should make sure that your child gets all of the recommended vaccines.

- Babies younger than 6 months cannot get the vaccine. Try to keep them away from people who show symptoms of influenza or a cold.

- Teach your child to clean his hands properly, especially after coughing, sneezing or wiping his nose or after being in contact with someone with the flu or a cold.

- Teach your children to cover their nose and mouth when they sneeze or cough.

- Teach your child to avoid sharing toys that young children place in their mouths until they are cleaned.

- Teach your child to avoid sharing cups, utensils or towels until they have been washed.

Chapter 8: Natural remedies against colds

Natural remedies are safe, help us to feel better, and, in most cases, are extremely cheap.

As a precaution, those recipes that include garlic or onion cannot be supplied to children younger than one and a half years old; while vapor rubs can be used on young children but only in the form of shower or baths.

Remedy 1: Chicken Soup (6 months and up)

Different scientific studies have shown that the chicken soup relieves cold symptoms like aches, fatigue, congestion, and fever as it has ingredients, like zinc and iron, which help against colds and influenza episodes.

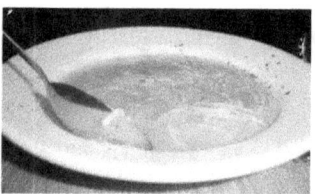

Besides, chicken soup has anti-inflammatory benefits able to reduce swellings and calm the skin around the nose.

Chicken Soup Recipe:
- 1 kilo of chicken in pieces
- 1 onion
- 1 carrot
- 1 leek
- Noodles for soup
- A pinch of mint
- 1 celery
- A pinch of chickpeas (optional)

25

- A pinch of salt

Directions:

- Clean the chicken and place it in a large cooking pot together with 1.5 liters of water, enough to cover the meat.

- Cut the carrot in two or three pieces and the onion in small pieces.

- Add the rest of the ingredients (carrot, onion, salt, celery, leek) to the pot and cook at a low temperature for two hours.

- Remove the chicken and the carrot and add the rest of the ingredients to the mixture.

- Add the crushed mixture to the water and cut the chicken and carrot into small pieces.

- Add some noodles, especially for soup.

- Add some chickpeas (optional).

- Serve warm.

Remedy 2: Honey (12 months and up)

Honey is a natural expectorant that helps eliminate mucus. Furthermore, thanks to its antiseptic benefits, honey is able to control and fight against throat infections.

These statements have been recently confirmed by a research project carried out at the Pennsylvania State University's College of Medicine. The study has shown that a teaspoon of honey before bedtime suppresses coughing significantly, while soothing throats in children between 2 and 5 years old. But you should be aware that children younger than one year old should not take honey, as it could cause a rare illness called infant botulism.

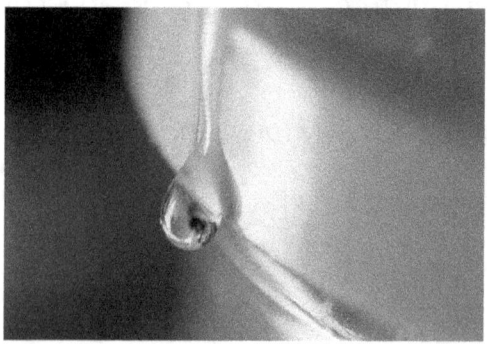

A good remedy consists of adding some honey in a glass of boiled water and pouring it into a bottle or container. Wait for about10 or 15 minutes until it is warm and add some squeezed lemon, which will provide vitamin C to the mixture.

For best results, gargle honey with a warm tea made with leaves of raspberries and two teaspoons of honey in half a cup of water. However, this remedy is not recommended for children younger than 4 because, although the mixture could be swallowed, the child can choke.

Remedy 3: Steamy air (all ages)

The humidity relieves the upper-airway swelling that can cause a croupy cough. Therefore, if your child has a cough, especially the kind known as croupy cough, which sounds like hacking or barking, run a hot, steamy shower and bring him into the bathroom; it will help open up his airways.

Simply, turn on the shower and let the hot water flow to allow the room to fill with steam. Then, close the bathroom door, block any gap under the door with a towel and sit the child in the steamy room for about 15 minutes, four times a day. The resulting warm air will help your child breathe more easily.

For children over the age of 2, adding a few drops of menthol to the bath water may also help the child feel less congested. You can purchase menthol oil at most natural food stores.

Remedy 4: The Power of Sleep (all ages)

A popular belief states, "Sleeping is the best medicine". It takes energy to fight an infection, and that can wear a child (or an adult) out. But when your child is resting, he is healing, which is exactly what he needs to do.

This is the perfect moment to let your child watch his favorite video or television program; bring him a new set of crayons and paper, a coloring book or a puzzle that can be manageable in bed. You can also bring him the phone so he can chat with the grandpas or a friend.

Make sure that your child does not spend all of his time in bed; as sometimes a change of scenery is helpful. If the weather is good, set up a comfortable place in the yard or on the porch for your child to rest. Indoors, fashion something more fun than his bed – like a tent in the living room or a snug, pillow-filled area near you.

Remedy 5: Saline Drops (all ages)

Drops clear the nose when kids are too young to blow their nose. For babies, a bulb syringe really comes in handy if a stuffy nose interferes with breastfeeding or bottle-feeding.

Clearing a stuffy nose with a bulb syringe works best for young babies. But if your older baby or child does not mind the procedure, there is no reason not to do it.

A homemade remedy consists in preparing saline drops at home by dissolving about 1/2 teaspoon of salt in 8 ounces of warm water. Make a fresh batch each day and store it in a clean, covered glass jar. Bacteria can grow in the solution; so do not keep it for more than 24 hours.

To apply the saline drops, you should follow the next steps:

1. Tip your child's head back or lay him on his back with a rolled-up towel supporting his head. Squeeze 2-3 drops of saline solution (1 drop in children younger than 12 months) into each nostril to thin and loosen the mucus. Try to keep the child's head still afterward for about 30 seconds (or less for a baby).

31

2. Squeeze the bulb of the syringe and gently insert the rubber tip into the nostril. Some doctors recommend also gently closing off the other nostril with your finger to get better suction from the bulb syringe.

3. Slowly release the bulb to collect mucus and saline solution.

4. Remove the syringe and squeeze the bulb to expel the mucus into a tissue.

5. Wipe the syringe and repeat with the other nostril.

6. Repeat the procedure, if necessary.

Bear in mind that you should not suction your child's nose more than a few times a day or you might irritate its lining and you should not use the saline drops for more than four days in a row, because they can dry out the child's nose over time.

If your child's nose is irritated or the baby is really upset by the syringe, just add a few drops of saline solution with a dropper and gently wipe the lower part of his nostrils with the help of a cotton swab, being careful not to insert the swab inside the nostrils.

You can also use the bulb syringe without saline to help remove mucus, by squeezing the bulb to force out air and gently inserting the tip in the nostril. Then, let the air out of the bulb to draw in mucus and remove the bulb and squeeze any mucus onto a tissue.

You can also use serum to clean the nose of a child or baby. The serum could be purchased in different sizes at any chemist.

A good tip is to warm the serum to adjust it to the temperature of the child's body, so the child does not feel very uncomfortable. The serum could be purchased in individual vials, which should never be introduced in the child's nostrils when applying it.

Spray products for children 2 and older are available at pharmacies without a prescription. However, doctors do not recommend them for young children, as nasal sprays are not very effective and can cause a rebound effect, making congestion worse in the long run because you can apply too much pressure and derive the mucus towards the throat and ears.

In the last years, nasal vacuums with interchangeable heads have reached the market. They could be bought at the chemists and should be used carefully; blowing gently or the pressure will derive mucus towards the child's ears and throat.

Remedy 6: Warm Liquids (all ages)

Warm liquids produce the same effect that a good chicken soup does in a weak body, lessening the symptoms of a cold.

With young children, the best thing to do is cut an apple into two halves and boil one of the halves in a bit of water, just enough to cover it. Then, squeeze the apple in the water and strain the mixture into a baby bottle or similar container and allow it to cool down a bit.

Another alternative for babies and young children is to give them some warm and weak chamomile tea. There are other herbal teas that are safe for children all ages but consult your doctor, as not all products are completely natural.

Warm liquids like roiboos can help children over the age of 5 to feel better, as they sooth cold's symptoms. Furthermore, the roiboos (which are flavored roots from South Africa) do not contain stimulants and strengthen the immune system.

Roiboos are completely natural and they can be found at any herb shops or supermarkets in a large range of flavors from chocolate to strawberry passing by orange, lemon or vanilla.

Remedy 7: The Cinnamon (2 years and up)

It is widely known that cinnamon has aphrodisiac effects. However, this is not completely true as it actually has stimulating effects, which is just what a weak body needs.

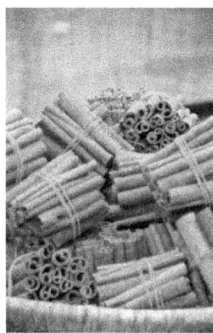

A good natural remedy that works like a wonder is to mix a bit a honey with some cinnamon until you get a paste, slightly thicker than syrup.

You could give the child a teaspoon of the mixture every three or four hours or, even better, stir your honey cinnamon mixture into a warm tea like chamomile or over fruit rich in vitamin C, like oranges, and the children use theirs as dip for fruit. To prepare the mixture you need just a 1-teaspoon of honey and 1/4 teaspoon of cinnamon.

Remedy 8: Eucalyptus Vapor Rubs (3 months and up)

Vapor rubs may help kids sleep better at night and, although some research projects have suggested that the ingredients used in the vapor rubs actually have no effect on nasal congestion, they make the cold sufferer feel better by producing a cooling sensation in the nose.

Vapor rubs can be massaged into your child's chest, neck, and/or back avoiding broken or sensitive skin and applying it to your child's mouth or nose, around the eyes, or anywhere on his face.

You can find vapor rub products made specifically for babies 3 months and older. This baby-safe version of the familiar commercial rub contains petrolatum, oils, and eucalyptus. It does not have camphor or menthol, which should not be used with children younger than 2 years old.

Natural vapor balms are also available, and are made of ingredients like aloe, herbs, oils, beeswax, and essential oils.

A homemade version is to add one or two drops of eucalyptus essential oil to one or two teaspoons of olive oil. Mix the ingredients throughout and rub them on the child's chest and neck or under his nose.

Remedy 9: Steamy Baths (2 years and up)

A steamy bath is one of the oldest and more effective natural remedies. You just have to boil some water and place it in a container; ask your child to place his head over the container with his eyes closed and a towel over his head so he can breathe the vapor produced by the boiling water. To avoid burns, be sure that your child does not approach the water too much and does not cover his entire head with the towel.

The vapor produced by the boiling water will help the child to breathe better and adding some eucalyptus, thyme or juniper to the water could boost the effect. Each session should last about 10 minutes and it's recommended that you do two daily sessions, one in the morning and another one at night.

If you child feels uncomfortable with the vapor (or he is younger than 2 years old) and he is not able to place his head under a towel, a soother version of this remedy consists of boiling some marjoram (adding one or two drops to a liter of water) and sit the child in the kitchen room, so he could breathe the vapor.

You can also buy herbal inhalers at the chemists. These products are safe for children and they are simple and easy to use. Your child can carry the inhaler in a pocket and inhale the scent to help him open his nose and lungs. Having their very own inhaler to carry around makes kids feel special—you could even let them decorate the jar if they are feeling up to it.

Children love having a choice, so you can let them pick the scent they would like to use, too. Some suggestions are: eucalyptus, mint, rosemary, and lavender.

Remedy 10: Plenty of Fluids (6 months and up)

Drinking plenty of fluids helps prevent dehydration and flushes and thins your child's nasal secretions. Therefore, it is recommended that you drink between 8 and 10 glasses of natural still water on a daily basis while avoiding stimulant beverages.

Plain water is great, but your child might not find it very appealing. Try fruit smoothies and other favorite healthful beverages, clear broths, soups, and herbal teas.

You should stick to breast or bottled milk for babies younger than 6 months old, unless your doctor allows you to offer him some weak chamomile tea, apple water or similar.

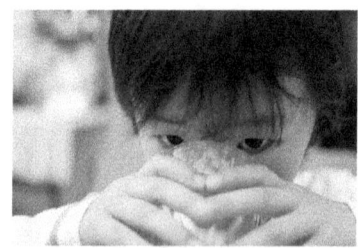

Remedy 11: Elevating the Head (12 months and up)

Elevating your child's head while he is resting can help him breathe more comfortably. Therefore, you should use towels or pillows to elevate the head of the mattress, or pillows to raise your toddler or older child's head.

If your child sleeps in a crib, place a couple of towels or a slim pillow underneath the head of the mattress on the crib springs. Do not try to raise the legs of the crib or you will make it unstable.

If your child sleeps in a big bed, an extra pillow under his head might do the trick but it is safer to raise the head of the bed by sliding towels or a pillow underneath the mattress. This also creates a more gradual, comfortable slope than extra pillows under the head.

For young babies, the best is letting your child sleep in his car seat as it usually could be reclined and the baby could rest better in a semi-upright position.

Remedy 12: Salted Water Gargling (4 years and up)

Gargling with salt water is a time-honored way to soothe a sore throat and helps clear mucus from the area. All that you need is some warm salt water. Simply, combine 1/2 teaspoon of salt in a glass of warm water and stir. If your child does not mind the taste, a squirt or two of fresh lemon juice can be a soothing addition.

Your child must be old enough to learn to gargle. For many kids, that means school age or older but some children can manage it sooner. Only have a younger child gargle if he is willing to learn and it makes him feel better. To start, the best solution is that your child practice with plain water. Ideally, your child should repeat the operation three or four times on a daily basis while feeling sick. But remember, that gargling is not recommended with very young children (younger than 4 or 5 years old).

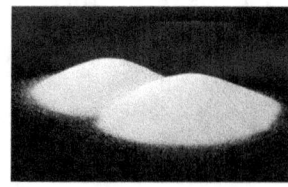

Remedy 13: Infusions (3 years and up)

Infusion 1: Add in some boiling water a teaspoon of bay, a teaspoon of cinnamon, and another teaspoon of sage.

Infusion 2: Make tea by boiling some water and adding a teaspoon of hot radish and plenty of honey to soothe the flavor. This tea works really well at the moment of fighting against chest congestion.

Infusion 3: Make a tea with 60 g of violets per liter of water. Let the mixture rest for 10 minutes, add 4 teaspoons of sugar and stir. Once the mixture is cold, strain and drink two or three times a day.

Infusion 4: Crush a piece of pomegranate peel and put it in a cup of boiled water, alongside with a pinch of mint and two fresh leaves of sage. Let the tea rest for 10 minutes, strain, soothe with honey, and drink two cups a day.

Infusion 5: Add a pinch of mint and a pinch of marshmallow to a cup of boiling water. Cover and let the mixture rest for 15 minutes before you strain it. Drink two cups a day.

Infusion 6: Boil a liter of water and add 10 g of basil. Cover, let it cool down and strain. Drink a glass a day with a bit a honey.

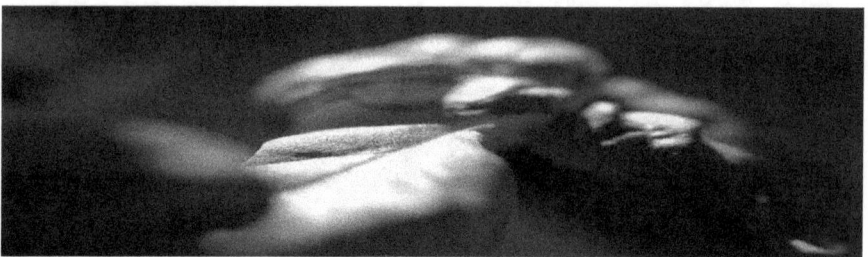

Infusion 7: Boil ½ a pot of water for 10 minutes with 7 leaves of cabbage and 3 stalks of leeks. Let the tea cool down and drink several glasses throughout the day. This remedy fights even the most resistant colds.

Infusion 8: Add 1 teaspoon of thyme to a cup of boiling water. Cover, strain, and let the tea cool down. Drink three times a day. This remedy is ideal for fighting colds, calming coughs, and soothing throats.

Infusion 9: Add a teaspoon of rosemary to a cup of water and let the mixture boil for 5 minutes. Let the tea cool down and drink three times a day.

Infusion 10: Boil a cup of water with a clove of garlic, a cave of cinnamon and a teaspoon of ginger in little pieces. Let the tea rest for 15 minutes, add a few drops of propolis and soothe the flavor with a teaspoon of honey.

Infusion 11: Boil 100 ml of water with 5 g of pennyroyal. Let the mixture cool down and drink three cups every day, preferably after meals.

Infusion 12: Add 2 teaspoons of thyme to a cup of boiling water. Cover and let it rest for around 10 minutes. Strain and add some honey and/or a bit of cinnamon. Drink three or four glasses on a daily basis to remove mucus.

Remedy 14: Milk (all ages)

Milk is a natural remedy against sore throats, although sometimes it can cause mucus.

If the child is a baby, maternal milk is the best option to reinforce the immune system.

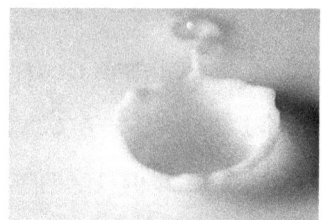

For children over 1 year old, a remedy against a cold is to add a teaspoon of butter and another teaspoon of honey to milk. Stir and add in the juice of a clove of garlic (optional), then; strain, and drink hot. You can also heat a cup of milk and add a teaspoon of butter and a pinch of black pepper.

Another version of this remedy consists of replacing the butter and the pepper with 1/2 teaspoon of dusted ginger and some honey.

Remedy 15: Mustard (12 months and up)

Mustard has expectorant effects and it could be prepared in the form of a rub to treat chest congestion. You have to mix in equal parts dry moustache and flour, making a paste with some warm water. The paste will be easier to remove after 10 or 15 minutes, if you massage some olive oil on the child's chest before applying the rub.

You can also prepare a tea based on mustard. Simply, cook some water at a low temperature for around 20 minutes, adding a teaspoon of grounded radish and another of mustard seeds. Then, strain the tea and add enough honey to form syrup that your child can drink twice a day.

Remedy 16: Garlic (2 years and up)

Garlic is one of the best natural anti-bacteria products, which is able to easily lessen the symptoms of a cold. Garlic is very effective against aches and throat irritations besides being an ally at the moment of combating a fever.

The best option is to eat garlic on its own but, let's face it, garlic is not the favorite condiment of children. You can familiarize your kids with its flavor by adding a bit to salads and vegetables or putting a couple of garlic cloves inside a bottle of oil to be used for salads.

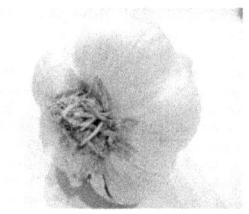

You can also keep a clove of garlic slightly beaten, or pierced with a fork, between the teeth and the interior of the cheek. After a while, throw away the garlic without eating it.

These remedies will not work very well with children. Therefore, the best option is that they swallow the clove of garlic with a bit of water, cutting it into little pieces if necessary.

Remedy 17: Salted Baths (4 years and up)

A salted bath flushes a mild saline solution through the nasal passages, moisturizing the area, which thin, loosens, and rinses away mucus.

You can simply fill a large bowl with some warm water, which has been previously boiled for 3 to 5 minutes or with distilled or sterile water available in stores. Then, add 1/2 teaspoon of salt to it and ask your child to introduce his face with their eyes closed. The idea is that some of the water enters the nostrils and cleans them.

You can also use a neti-pot to take this operation on board. A neti-pot looks like a very small watering can or teapot, which are typically ceramic or metal. You can buy neti-pots at drugstores, natural food stores or online. By tilting your child's head sideways over the sink and placing the spout of the pot in the top nostril, you can run water through the nasal passages to clean and moisturize them while your child breathes through his mouth. This takes a little trial and error, being recommended to first try on yourself before teaching your child to use the neti pot.

Your child must be old enough and willing to go along with the procedure, which is not painful but does feel strange at first. This remedy does not work with babies or young toddlers and always remember not to force a child who is not interested.

Remedy 18: Onion (12 months and up)

Alongside the garlic, the onion is the best natural product against colds and influenza episodes, and the star in any anti-cold diet. The best thing to do is eat some onion by itself, but this usually does not work with children who refuse its taste.

A solution is to make onion syrup with a large onion, some sugar, and a bit of honey (optional). Cut the onion in small pieces and place them in a bowl, adding some teaspoons of sugar. Then, let the onion rest for a few hours to allow the sugar to extract the juice of the onion. The liquid should be strained and drunk three or four times on a daily basis, preferably after meals. This remedy has expectorant and disinfectant effects, working especially well on the throat.

You can also prepare a delicious onion soup to decongest the respiratory track. This soup has the same effects that a chicken soup does and you can add some chicken to facilitate the meal for children.

Another traditional remedy is to place one or several onions, cut in pieces, on the bedside table in order to favor decongestion and calm coughs.

Finally, try vapor inhalations by cutting and boiling a large onion in half a liter of water. Then, place the container in the child's room to allow steam to clean the respiratory track.

Remedy 19: Chamomile (all ages)

Chamomile is an herb that has numerous health benefits and it is used to help with a wide range of illnesses.

The best remedy consists of adding two tea bags of chamomile to a liter of boiling water and breathing the steam for around 5 minutes (young babies and toddlers) or 10 minutes (older children).

You can also use a bit of that tea to be absorbed with the help of a dropper and introduce a couple of drops on each of the child's nostrils.

The chamomile tea can also be used to wet a piece of cotton and clean the exterior of the child's nose to obtain a calming effect on the irritated areas.

Some doctors recommend giving a bottle with some weak chamomile to babies who are fighting a cold but always make sure to consult your doctor when the child is very young.

Remedy 20: Vitamin C (12 months and up)

Vitamin C is the "king" of all vitamins, which is able to reinforce the immune system to help the body fight against the symptoms of colds and influenza.

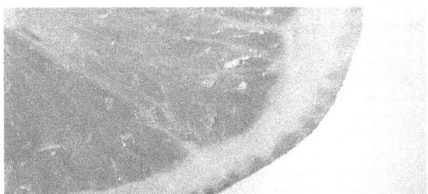

There are chewable vitamin C capsules for children available at the chemists and also in stores.

Regarding natural products, those containing a higher dose of vitamin C are vegetables and fruits, especially citric fruits. You can prepare a juice with a cup of water, two oranges, a lemon, and a teaspoon of honey.

Another drink that is rich in vitamin C and has anti-bacteria benefits is obtained with the following ingredients: 20 ml of garlic juice, a cup of orange juice, and a pineapple slice. Add all the ingredients in the mixture for three minutes and drink the juice.

One more drink with that contains high levels of vitamin C is carrot juice. To soothe its flavor for the children, you can mix it with some apple and/or orange juice.

At the first sign of a cold, dose your kid up with vitamin C— oranges, carrots, chewable vitamins- that will help boost his immune system and shorten the duration of a cold.

Remedy 21: Foot Massages (12 months and up-consult with your doctor regarding younger children)

The massages do not contribute to eliminate the virus but they relax the patient's body making him feel better and lessening the ache.

The massages should be given on the foot plants on a daily basis. For the massage, use around 15 drops of tea tree essential oil, this will help to release the pain related to the cold process.

Remedy 22: Juices and Smoothies (12 months and up)

Milkshakes, juices, and smoothies are essential in any cold episode as, besides keeping the body moisturized, they offer the necessary vitamins to help the immune system fight against infections.

Use one of the following recipes to help your child feel better during a cold process. You can add some milk to juice to obtain a milkshake.

Tomato Juice: Add in a blend, a cup of water, 3 medium tomatoes in pieces, a bunch of parsley, a small piece of celery, 1/3 cucumber in pieces, one clove of garlic, and two slices of onion (add some sugar or honey to soothe the flavor). Drink a glass twice a week before breakfast.

Carrot Juice: Wash and mix 2 carrots, 1/2 bunch of radish, 1/2 bunch of spinach, 2 small pieces of celery, the juice of two lemons, and a glass of water. This juice should be drunk for a week before breakfast.

Strawberry Juice: Add a cup of strawberries with 1/2 cup of apples, a cup of sliced bananas, a teaspoon of honey, and a cup of water. Mix all the ingredients to form a paste and drink every morning for a week. If the liquid is too dense, add a bit of water or milk.

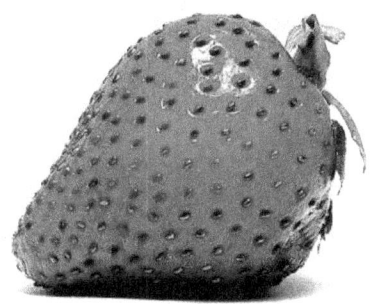

Apple Juice: Wash and peel two large apples, cut them into small pieces and place them in a cooking pot covering the apples with water. Cook the apples for around one hour at a low temperature and strain the water. The resulting juice should be allowed to cool down before drinking.

Remedy 23: Lemon (12 months and up)

The lemon is a natural source of vitamin C and a powerful ally against colds, influenza, and bronchitis thanks to its anti-virus and anti-inflammatory properties. This fruit is anti-bacteria and antiseptic, containing a great deal of flavonoids that protect respiratory channels and reinforce the benefits of the vitamin C. The lemon is easy to give to children in the form of refreshing lemonade.

A good remedy is to squeeze the juice of three lemons and add it to some boiling water. Add six or seven teaspoons of honey and a clove of garlic (if your child can stand the flavor) to boost the anti-bacteria and expectorant effects. Let the mix rests for 24 hours and strain it. Give three large spoons of the drink to your child during the cold process. The rest of the year, you can give your child a spoon of this tea to prevent future colds or influenza. You can also prepare hot tea by adding the juice and a bit of the peel of a lemon to a large glass of water. Boil the water for 10 minutes and let it cool down. Then, add some honey to soothe the flavor and drink the tea while still warm three times a day.

Remedy 24: Leek (12 months and up)

The leek shares many benefits with garlic and onion with the advantage of having a sweeter and more delicate flavor. The leek is rich in selenium (a stimulant of the immune system) and it contains a great dose of vitamins C and E, both of them with a high level of anti-oxidants.

The leek contributes to calm the symptoms of laryngitis and pharyngitis, as well as bronchitis and aphonia.

As the flavor of the leek is not the favorite of a child, you can offer it in soups mixing the leek with carrots and potatoes.

Remedy 25: Ginger (12 months and up)

Ginger, just like onion, is the star product in any influenza or cold process. In fact, a recent study developed by the prestigious medical association "Archives of Family Medicine" in the United States, has concluded that ginger has analgesic and anti-bacteria properties.

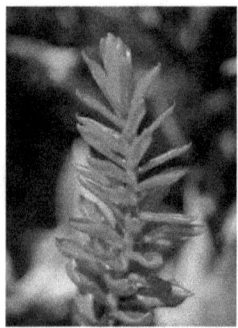

To calm the discomfort caused by a cold, it is a good idea to prepare a tea smashing a teaspoon of fresh ginger and adding it to a cup of boiling water. You can add a bit of honey to soothe the flavor and the juice of a natural lemon to provide some vitamin C.

Another option is to prepare a ginger tea boiling a piece of ginger in some water to clean colds' stuffy noses and calm coughs. Add a little honey or sugar to sweeten it up for kids.

Remedy 26: The Elderflower (2 years and up)

The elderflower has the same effects as a natural aspirin, being able to release pains and fight against a fever. Besides, the elderflower has sambucol, a natural ingredient that combats the infection caused by the influenza.

The elderflower relaxes the body and it could be drunk as a hot tea. Simply, add a teaspoon of grounded bark and berries in boiling water and let the liquid rest for 10-15 minutes, then; strain and drink three times a day, preferably after meals.

Remedy 27: Camphor Rubs (2 years and up)

The camphor has calming effects thanks to its analgesic properties, while it is able to lessen skin irritation thanks to its antiseptic benefits.

The camphor could be applied as rubs that could be purchased at any natural shop or chemist.

To obtain better results, you can add a few drops of eucalyptus to the rub or buy a rub that contains both ingredients. In this way, the child could benefit not only from the analgesic properties of the camphor but also from the expectorant effects of the eucalyptus. The rub should be applied on the neck, chest, and/or back of the child, being very careful of avoiding mouth, eyes, and nose.

If the child's nose is irritated, you can apply a bit of this rub under the nose but being careful that it does not reach the interior of the nostrils. This remedy only works with children over the age of six or seven who could be careful and avoid contact with eyes, mouth, and nose.

Remedy 28: Echinacea (2 years and up)

Echinacea is a root with powerful medical properties able to reinforce and stimulate the immune system to help it fight against infections and viruses. It can be found in natural shops and chemists in the form of tablets or as a solution. Maybe for children, the best is to get a solution and add some drops (following the instructions on the package) to juices and milkshakes.

Some research projects claim that taking Echinacea at the beginning of a cold can cut it off while other studies claim that it serves to lessen the duration of a cold. In fact, the Echinacea is not only able to reduce the effects of a cold but it can also prevent it, if taken regularly.

As it is a natural product, the Echinacea protects and strengthens the body against future infections. However, many doctors discourage the continuous use of Echinacea in children.

Remedy 29: The Pleasure of Food (all ages)

Children, in general, have few or no appetite when sick because the infection reduces the capability of the body to ingest food. Therefore, do not force you child to eat if he does not feel like.

During a cold, you should avoid sugar and food with high levels of fat like frites, hamburgers, hot-dogs, chocolates, pastries or peanut butter, as the body would derive resources to the digestion instead of concentrating on fighting against the infection. Replace that kind of food with flour, chicken soup, jelly, fruits or apple compote, easier to eat and more nutritive.

Also, you should avoid excessively cold or hot food that could irritate the throat and slow down the child's recovery.

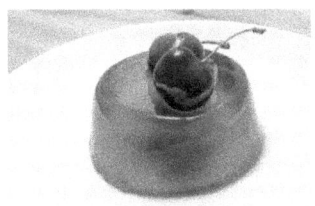

Remedy 30: Physical Activity (all ages)

When the child starts feeling better, it is recommended to combine periods of rest with some physical activity or games. These activities should be developed, preferably, in the interior of the house to avoid drastic changes of temperature or airflows.

The exercise will help the child to find an entertainment and to liberate mucus easily. Physical activity also contributes to reinforce the natural defenses of the body and to sleep better as the child will feel more tired.

Remedy 31: Propolis (2 years and up)

Propolis is a natural product extracted by the bees from the buds of the trees, being able to reinforce and protect the defenses of our immune system.

During the cold, a few drops of propolis will reinforce the immune system, shortening the duration of the cold process by acting as a natural antibiotic.

You can add a few drops of propolis to juices and milkshakes to soothe the flavor, which could be too bitter for children.

Remedy 32: Smacks in the Back (all ages)

A remedy very often used on children with colds is simply place the child on your lap and palm his back carefully.

You should lean your child on your lap in a 30° angle and, then, scoop your hand and carefully palm the back of the child.

This remedy is recommended especially in babies, who cannot be offered most of the remedies explained in this book.

Remedy 33: Relaxing Baths (all ages)

One of the most popular natural remedies against a cold is a relaxing bath in a steamy room.

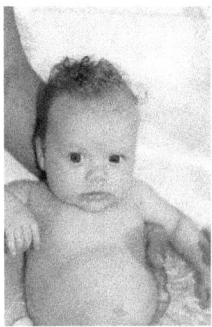

Simply, let the shower run for a few minutes to produce vapor and then submerge your child in a warm bath but measuring the temperature of the water to avoid burns. If the child is old enough, let him play in the bath as long as he likes while you supervise.

Breathing moist air helps loosen the mucus in the nasal passages while a warm bath has the added benefit of relaxing your child.

If the child is older than one year, you can add a few drops of lavender essential oil to boost the relaxing effects or a few drops of eucalyptus oil to increase the expectorant effects.

Remedy 34: Menthol Rubs (2 years and up)

Massaging a bit of menthol under the nose of your child can help him breathe easier can also relieve irritated skin.

You can make your own rub by heating a cup of oil such as olive oil or coconut oil (or a mix;) and 1/4 cup beeswax in a double boiler over low heat until the beeswax is melted. Then pour into containers and add 10-20 drops of eucalyptus essential oil while it is still warm.

Once the salve cools and thickens, if you want to adjust the thickness of the salve, simply heat it again and add more beeswax. Apply the rub on the chest, back, and/or neck.

You can also experiment with adding other essential oils, such as lavender to boost the relaxing effects.

Remedy 35: Cold Poultices (all ages)

When the child coughs too much, you can help him by placing cold compresses with poultices.

The poultices that obtain the best results are made with cottage cheese or potatoes. You should place a dressing on the chest of the child and put some cooked and smashed potatoes or one-centimeter layer of cottage cheese. You can also wrap potatoes or cottage cheese in a light towel and place it on the chest and/or back of the child.

The poultice will act as a disinfectant of the breathing system, providing a pleasant and releasing effect. But be careful that the potatoes are not too hot in order to avoid burns.

Remedy 36: Against Dry Cough (12 months and up)

A dry cough is one of the most common symptoms of any cold and influenza and it could result in being extremely irritated and uncomfortable.

To reduce the symptoms of a cold, you could use lemon juice and olive oil. The vitamins found in lemons and the multiple benefits of olive oils in the body, will be successful in calming coughs and reinforcing the immune system.

Simply, mix 200 ml of olive oil to the juice of one lemon. Then, shake and give the child a large spoon three times a day. For the best results, you can add a bit of honey to soothe the throat and calm the cough almost immediately.

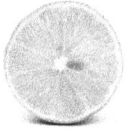

Remedy 37: Against Wet Cough (2 years and up)

Wet cough could be fought in different ways without medicine. A good solution is to prepare a tea made of honey and onions. You just have to chop three onions and add a half glass of honey, stirring the mix and let the tea rest for around 3 hours. After this time, boil 50 ml of water and add it to the mixture. Let the tea cool down for about three hours and strain the resulting juice. Give the child a teaspoon of this tea several times a day.

Another effective remedy is the fennel syrup, obtained by adding a teaspoon of fennel seeds to 1/3 liter of water. Then, add 2 teaspoons of honey and let the tea cook for around 10 minutes. Strain the tea and drink three times a day, warm or cold.

Remedy 38: Against the Fever (all ages)

The appearance of fever is a sign that the body is fighting against the infection.

The fever produces sweating and a loss of hydration in the body. Therefore, drinking plenty of fluids is vital to help the body fight against the virus. You should give the child herb and fruit teas, juices, smoothies, milkshakes, and water up to a total of 2 liters of liquid a day. Another option is to prepare a good chicken or onion soup and serve hot.

Besides, you should check the temperature and humidity of the child's room constantly to make sure that the area is not very hot or dry and it can provoke a lack of hydration in the breathing channels and the possibility that the virus will reproduce and spread.

Make sure that the child is covered only by light-weight blankets or something similar that still allows heat to escape and that he does not have problems breathing.

The best remedy against a fever is to use light clothing (preferably just underwear) to allow the body to release heat.

If the fever increases, a good remedy is to give the child a rather cold shower or bath.

Another alternative, is trying cold compresses, which should be applied on the child's forehead, neck, nape, and the interior parts of the calves. Cold compresses produce a calming effect and release the heat caused by the fever.

You can also fill a sink or basin with lukewarm water, and use a washcloth to gently wipe over the body.

Remedy 39: Against Ear Pain (all ages)

One of the most efficient remedies against ear pains is a compress made with onions, which are able to reduce the inflammation in the hearing channel.

Simply, place a chopped onion in a small cotton bag and heat the bag with the help of vapor. Place the bag on the damaged ear and cover it with a handkerchief.

Another traditional remedy consists of folding fabric handkerchiefs and heating them with the help of an iron to then place them on the ear.

Finally, consult your doctor or take your child to the hospital if he complains of intense pain or you believe that his ear is infected.

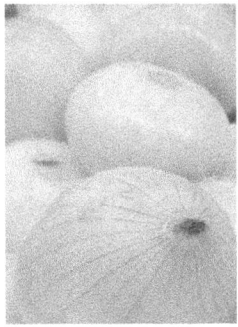

Remedy 40: Against Sore Throats (all ages, except gargling)

A good remedy to calm sore throats is placing a compress on the neck of the child to obtain instant calming effects.

For the dressing, you can use quark (cottage cheese) or potatoes and prepare it in the same way that cold poultices explained in remedy 35.

As previously mentioned, an alternative to calming a sore throat is the salted gargling (make sure that your child is old enough and can do them without swallowing the water or chocking).

Finally, remember to offer plenty of warm drinks and a good chicken or onion soup, which is rich in zinc and iron. Do not forget that hot drinks are very useful in cases of pharyngitis, tonsillitis or sore throats.

Index of Illustrations

1. Sneeze. Author: Futurestreet on www.flickr.com license creative.commons atribution 2.0 generic.

2. School. Author: Andres Ruff Custom Designs on www.flickr.com licence creative.commons atribution 2.0 generic.

3. Wash your Hands. Author: Miki Yoshihito on www.flickr.com licence creative.commons atribution 2.0 generic.

4. Flu. Author: Futureatlas.com on www.flickr.com license creative.commons atribution 2.0 generic.

5. Chicken Soup. Author: Shawn Rossi on www.flickr.com license creative.commons atribution 2.0 generic.

6. Honey. Author: Dino Giordano on www.flickr.com license creative.commons atribution 2.0 generic.

7. Cinnamon. Author: Vvillamon on www.flickr.com license creative.commons atribution 2.0 generic.

8. Drinking Water. Author: Akihito Fujii on www.flickr.com license creative.commons atribution 2.0 generic.

9. Salt. Author: SoraZG on www.flickr.com license creative.commons atribtion 2.0 generic.

10. Basil. Author: Gonzalo MMD on www.flickr.com license creative.commons atribution 2.0 generic.

11. Milk. Author: Tambako the Jaguar on www.flickr.com license creative.commons atribution 2.0 generic.

12. Garlic. Author: Lowjumpingfrog on www.flickr.com license creative.commons atribution 2.0 generic.

13. Orange. Author: DavidDennisPhotos on www.flickr.com, creative.commons atribution 2.0 generic.

14. Strawberry. Author: Bdebaca on www.flickr.com license creative.commons atribution 2.0 generic.

15. Ginger. Author: Waywuwei on www.flickr.com license creative.commons atribution 2.0 generic.

16. Jelly. Author: Mordicua on www.flickr.com license creative.commons atribution 2.0 generic.

17. Relaxing Bath. Author: Joe Shlabotnik on www.flickr.com license creative.commons atribution 2.0 generic.

18. Lemon. Author: Bdebaca on www.flickr.com license creative.commons atribution 2.0 generic.

19. Onions. Author: Vacacion on www.flickr.com license creative.commons atribution 2.0 generic.